Beyond the Fear of Stuttering

My Journey to Self Acceptance and Freedom

Mary Wood

Contents

To request permissions, contact the publisher at dmarywood@yahoo.com.

Paperback ISBN: 9798431504518

Cover, formatting, and book production by Michael Lacey with Story Builds Creative (affiliate links through Amazon Associates).

Story-Builds.com

First paperback edition March 2021.

FOREWORD

I've been attending stuttering association conferences in Canada and the US for many years now and I always seek out and attend Mary Wood's inspirational workshops and keynote speeches. Not only does she draw a good-sized crowd consistently, but she has an amazing talent to get everyone actively involved sharing their stories, emotions, and opinions, and often bringing 'AHA!' moments to participants. She is welcoming, open and wise, offering advice about life that can help everyone, not just those who stutter! "Who would you be and what would you do in someone else's presence without the story that they should care about or love you?" Mary asks, and the response from a participant is: "This would be SO LIBERATING!" . That is Mary's inspiration in action! "I love myself the way I am! There's nothing I need to change" are words she shares from a favourite song. That's an affirmation for all! Many of us can agree that we love Mary, just the way she is! Mary Wood IS LOVE! I am grateful for Mary's teaching and message and for her support and wisdom to the stuttering community. I guarantee that this book contains important information, inspiration and opportunity for personal and spiritual growth for us all.

Eeva Stierwalt, National Coordinator and Chair
Canadian Stuttering Association

Mary's generosity and willingness to meet me, at the time a complete stranger, changed my life. My view and therefore my path in life shifted. Her willingness to seek truth and love at the deepest of levels are guiding. I am very grateful for her influence.

Kim Block: Author of "A Stuttering Superhero"

I spent the first 50 years of life consumed by shame about my stuttering and living in fear of rejection by others because of my stuttering. At a workshop at the 2010 National Stuttering Association conference, Mary taught us about accepting what is, and loving what is. It's not about not stuttering, as that is what causes the shame and the fear in the first place, but rather it's about accepting and embracing reality, especially when it is uncomfortable, and from there finding our way to survive and thrive. I am forever grateful to Mary for showing me the way then and for continuing to teach me over the years. I encourage you to read this book, find the lessons that benefit you, and then reread it, as our minds change over time and perhaps open up to new ideas.

Hanan Hurwitz, Quality Management Consultant, ISAD committee member, and past Executive Director of The Israeli Stuttering Association

Mary is one of those people who come into your life and never leaves - but in the most impactful way. My own journey of acceptance and facing my fears started when I met Mary and attended her workshops. When I first heard the teachings of Mary, it changed my life. She made me look at my life and the people around me in a new light. She taught me to look inside of myself and face the fears that had been preventing me from doing all the things. We became very close ever since and I consider her one of my dearest friends. I am the person I am today in part because of Mary's workshops and her warm loving approach to life.

David Block, member of the Canadian Stuttering Association

The world of a stutterer can be a dark, lonely place. Mary Wood is a beacon of hope for those gripped in fear. For the past few decades, Mary has presented life altering events that enable stutterers to break free of self defeatism and begin living their best life. She uses her intuitive manner to unearth what's hidden in a person's psyche, initiating self understanding and healing. Her workshops are often the highlight of stuttering support conferences worldwide. Mary's work is a must-read for people who stutter!

Tom Scharstein

Chairman of the Board | worldstutteringnetwork.net | worldstutteringnetwork@gmail.com

When Mary speaks about stuttering, she speaks from the depths of her being. Through a process of deep and honest reflection on her experiences as a person who stutters, Mary found self-love and peace, and passionately set out to help others who also stutter. Mary's warmth and openness, and her messages of understanding, compassion, acceptance, love, and forgiveness have touched, influenced, brought hope, and inspired thousands of persons who stutter. Mary is "one of a kind", and a gift to the stuttering community.

Carla Di Domenicantonio, M.H.Sc.

Speech Language Pathologist and Friend

From the first time I met Mary back in 1994 at a National Stuttering Conference in Cleveland Ohio, I knew she was going to be a special person in my life.

She became more than just a friend; she became a mentor. She embodied the positive attitude I was working on, was joyful, so interesting and most importantly, had a genuineness that had you seeking her out for words of wisdom and guidance.

I am so happy that others will have the opportunity to learn from Mary as she shares her words, her life story and encourages others to take their own journey to find their own inner peace and self-awareness.

Annie Bradberry

Former National Stuttering Association Executive Director

CHAPTER 1
───────

AND SO MY JOURNEY BEGINS...

January 21, 1989 is a day I will always remember. I attended a Bob Proctor Seminar entitled "Born Rich" in Toronto. From the title I thought it was all about money. I was a single Mom at the time and could use some financial advice, but this was not where I would get it. Instead, the workshop was focused on how my mind works in conjunction with my thoughts.

I had stuttered for almost 50 years, and I knew that this information would change my life. I left the workshop with these words ringing in my ears:

"The mind controls the body. What I think about I bring about."

Then on the way home, more words came to me:

"I don't have to stutter anymore."

Even though I didn't really understand what these words meant, I believed them and knew they would bring change to my life. Little did I know to what extent.

I discovered later that I'd always been a covert stutterer – finding thousands of ways to hide it. I think I began stuttering when I was about three years old. My father stuttered too, but we never talked about it. It was always something that just seemed to be there. He died when he was 80 years old, and I often wonder how he felt about "it." I really wish that we had brought it out of the closet, told each other how we felt, and how we could help each other.

The first time I was aware of stuttering was in kindergarten when, sitting in a circle on the floor, we were asked to tell the colours of wool in a basket. I couldn't say the word "blue." Something didn't feel good to me as I saw the looks on the other kid's faces. When I was in public school, I can remember being with my friends and writing what I wanted to say on a small blackboard because I was afraid to speak. Mom would send me to the grocery store around the corner with a list of what she wanted, so I didn't have to speak.

Mom took me to speech therapy. The only time I can remember I was standing in a big room and reading Shakespeare's writing from a big book. I know that she was doing what she thought best and what was available at the time.

All through public school and high school, no one else who stuttered showed up in my life. In high school, I decided to be a secretary, taking the commercial course because I thought there was no way I could go to a university where I would have to speak in front of others. In shorthand class, the teacher by-passed me when she was going alphabetically through the class for student answers. Even though I liked this in one way, in another way it made me feel ashamed and different.

When I was asked for my name, I would often say Mary Smith because I knew I didn't stutter on s's – not very original, was it! I can remember my first day at work as a secretary at The Steel Company of Canada. There was a phone on my desk that I was expected to answer – omg! – I guess I always expected someone else was going to look after that part of the job! I worked in the Sales Department, and "S" was a good beginning sound for me so that worked most of the time. And when it didn't work, then I answered with a beginning "Ummm" which led me to begin what I needed to say.

This is the first time I have thought about this in many years, and a smile comes as I remember the people and the many happy days I spent there. After almost 30 years, I left the Steel Company, and moved on to the Hamilton Region Conservation Authority where I worked as an Administrative Assistant with the woman who invited me to the Bob Proctor Seminar that changed my life.

I attended the "Born Rich" seminar six times ... and each time came away with something different. This information was new to me and I wanted to understand all that I could because I knew it would change how I dealt with stuttering.

After my second time at the seminar, I spoke to Bob Proctor, told him I was a person who stuttered and he gave me these words as an affirmation (positive words that you repeat to change your beliefs): "I am so happy now that I can relax and my speech is fluent." So every day I would repeat these words – in the shower, in my car, when I got up in the morning, before I went to bed. I was slowly changing my beliefs about me as a person who stutters.

In my earlier '30s, I found a Speech Language Pathologist (SLP) in Toronto and my eyes were opened to a new kind of therapy. This was the first time the topic of fear around stuttering was put into words. There were eight of us in the group. Every week, we went to the mall with another person from the group and had a list of questions that we asked people about stuttering – what they thought and felt and knew about "it." My partner was "Wild Bill" – an older-then-I-was man with a good sense of humour.

A whole new world was opening up, and even though it was a scary one, it felt right ... and in some ways exciting. It was also the first time I sat with other people who stutter, heard their experiences, and could relate. At this point, I hadn't heard about self-help or support groups.

Through association with the Proctor group, I was introduced to a book by Napoleon Hill, *Think and Grow Rich* (another book I thought was about money) that lists our main fears. The first two were Fear of Poverty and Fear of Rejection. The fear of rejection...

Wow, I didn't have to continue on the list to know this was the fear that was such a large part of my life. More on this in the chapter entitled "Fear." I'm smiling as I'm thinking "and where else would it be?"

In 1992, I went to a support group meeting in Toronto for people who stutter. I can't remember what led me there. Another new world was opening and I dove in with both feet. This was a group of people I could listen and relate to, and then have them listen to my thoughts and experiences. It was through this group that I was introduced to CAPS, the Canadian Association for People Who Stutter – now changed to the CSA – Canadian Stuttering Association.

It was Ottawa 1993, which was the first self-help conference I attended where I met more understanding, kind, compassionate, and sometimes funny people. I had submitted a workshop proposal, and they accepted it. I still can't remember where the courage came from to do that. My sister Janet came with me for moral support. There were so many people who I could relate to, who I felt understood what I was feeling; people who became my life-long friends. From that conference, another new organization was introduced – the National Stuttering Association in the U.S.A.

The first NSA conference I went to was in Cleveland in 1994. And it was there that I learned another important awareness. For years I thought I stuttered because my Dad stuttered. I thought it was hereditary. For many years I had watched Dad not answering the phone, asking Mom to make telephone calls for him, so I thought this was what it was going to be like for me for the rest of my life. These words do not come from anger, but from acceptance, knowing Dad was doing the best he could do.

But I was beginning to question this…is there something else, some reason? Where did the stuttering really begin? John Harrison, author and long-time member of the NSA, presented a workshop at this conference and said that stuttering can be caused by wanting to emulate someone, wanting to copy them. When he said that, I realized what I think I knew and had been questioning – I emulated my father so that he would love me. After the workshop was over, I stood in the line to thank John for his workshop and for what I considered a very important life-changing realization. When I was standing in front of him, tears of gratitude came and I gave him a great big slobbery hug…whether he wanted it or not. I couldn't say anything for a minute or two. Here was this woman whom he had never met before, crying and hanging on to him, before uttering a single word. We often laughed about that after I introduced myself and explained the reason for the "assault."

This conference in Cleveland was the first of many more conferences in the United States, Canada, England, Germany, and Belgium. Many friendships that were made along the way still continue today, with many opportunities to learn more about stuttering, about who I really am. So many opportunities to love and serve, to laugh, to travel – the gifts just kept coming and still do.

Those are just a few of my first memories of stuttering. Then, on that day 50 years later, I began a journey that was first focused on fluency — and then changed to self-acceptance along the way. Both sides of this journey are in the pages that follow. At times, the stories and experiences may be repeated in different chapters as one relates to another. They overlap for me. It is a journey that still continues today, and I share with you some ideas that have opened my mind and heart along the way. I invite you to take out of them whatever you want, whatever feels right for you. My hope is that my experience in some way will let you realize how truly awesome you are!

CHAPTER 2

THOUGHTS

"What I think about I bring about."

These words from the Proctor seminar have changed my life in many ways. What I'm thinking about shows up in my world. From these words, I came to realize that stuttering was a self-fulfilling prophecy for me. That was an awesome awareness! When I answered the phone, there was this thought, this little voice that said, "Mary, you're going to stutter." In fact, every time I spoke, that thought was there. I came to realize that my thoughts do manifest in my world. Such a powerful understanding that changed and still continues to change my life in so many ways!

Realizing what I am thinking about and how important that is has been an important part of this journey, and still continues to be. Positive and loving thoughts attract positive and loving circumstances into our lives. Negative thoughts attract negative circumstances into our lives. Positive thoughts empower us – negative thoughts weaken our ability to perform.

Here's what I found on the internet relating to our thoughts. "In 2005, the National Science Foundation published an article summarizing research on human thoughts per day. It was found that the average person has about 12,000 to 60,000 thoughts per day. Of those thousands of thoughts, *80% were negative, and 95% were exactly the same repetitive thoughts as the day before.* We can see that one of the tendencies of the mind is to focus on the negative and 'play the same songs' over and over again." (I still need to remember that today!)

There was another interesting study (Leahy, 2005, Study of Cornell University) in which scientists found that the first 85% of what we worry about never happens. Second, with the 15% of the worries that did happen, 79% of the subjects discovered that either they could handle the difficulty better than expected or the difficulty taught them a lesson worth learning.

Below is an exercise you might like to do at a support meeting that shows how powerful our thoughts are and what effect they have on our strength and physiology.

Hold your arm out straight, as strong as you can make it. Now say "my name is" and repeat your own name. Now try to push your arm down. It's difficult to move. Now say "my name is" and repeat someone else's name. Now try to push your arm down. Your arm goes down easy.

When you tell a lie, you briefly disorient your brain and this affects your strength and physiology. We get the same results when we tell ourselves negative things and visualize negative pictures and outcomes.

Susan Jeffers' book *What to Say When You Talk to Yourself* really helped me understand how this thought process works. Our self talk (what we say when we talk to ourselves) depends on our programming – the thoughts we've sent to our subconscious mind over many years. The subconscious mind is listening and waiting for instructions. It doesn't care what we tell it – it just follows orders. Isn't that awesome... and a little scary at the same time?

Our thoughts and programming then create beliefs, beliefs create attitudes, attitudes create feelings, feelings determine actions, and actions create results. You might have to read that sentence a couple of times to understand what's going on – I know I did! It has been said that our attitude is either 90% of our solution or 90% of our problem. So, do you think it would be a good idea to include attitudinal therapy along with speech therapy?

We can change our thoughts and programming through affirmations that are positive statements we say to ourselves. It is said that after saying an affirmation for 30 days, we own it. I'd like to share a couple of my favourites with you ... ones I said many times a day very often for a lot more than 30 days. I said them in the morning before I went to work, when I was driving in my car, and before I went to bed. It helps if we repeat these while looking at ourselves in a mirror. That can feel a little weird and scary at first.

#1 on my hit parade is "I am love, I am joy, I am enough." I didn't know I was enough, and thought I needed someone else to make me feel good. Just nine little words that have made such a difference in my life. I'd say these while looking at myself in the mirror — and my kids thought I had lost it! I'm still repeating this affirmation to this day.

Here are some if you're focused on fluency:

"I am so happy now that I am relaxed and my speech is fluent." (That came from Bob Proctor.)

"Every day in every way I am getting better and better."

"No matter what you say or do to me, I am still a worthwhile person."

Our worth is established by the fact that we are here. You and I are all winners! Why? Because we won the greatest race of all – the sperm race! When we were conceived, 50 million sperm were racing to reach that egg – and you and I won! There are no losers – only winners! (Tee hee)

Then we entered the real world. We listened to what people told us we should do, who we should be, how we should think (if we were taught to think at all), and how we should speak. Wow! Look at all those "should's." Now we have an opportunity to change this programming because most of it isn't ours - it is somebody else's.

As I write this, it is almost 33 years since I heard the words "what I think about I bring about" for the first time and they are still a major lesson and awareness for me. They are also part of the groundwork in the chapters that follow. Thank you for being on this journey with me.

Chapter 3

Fear

Let's begin with a couple of definitions of fear:

- F.E.A.R. Fantasized Experience Appearing Real.
- Fear: Faith that the wrong thing is going to happen.

You and I have might have our own definition of fear – not what's above – but I know that fear has been my enemy at times and also my lesson. It still continues to be some days. Many times, fear controls us rather than you and I controlling it. But fear has also been a motivator for me after I took the time to understand where it comes from, and how I can move through it and past it.

Napoleon Hill, in his book *Think and Grow Rich* , said that before we can master an enemy, we must know its name, its habits and its place of abode. So I invite you to spend some time with me as we begin to understand what fear is, why it is at times a large part of who we are, acknowledging it, and accepting it as we learn to live with it, and grow with it. Grow with it, you say… now that was something new for me!

Let's start with the 6 Basic Fears that are listed in the first chapter of Napoleon Hill's book:

1. The fear of poverty.
2. The fear of criticism.
3. The fear of ill health.
4. The fear of Loss of Love.
5. The fear of age.
6. The fear of dying.

What do you think our main fear is as People Who Stutter (PWS)? When I read this list, the fear of criticism (or rejection) jumped off the page. Wow – I had found my #1 fear. Many years ago, I can remember reading a quote by Wendell Johnson, formerly a Professor of Speech Pathology at the University of Iowa, "There is no stuttering where there is no fear of stuttering." Now there are some words that made me stand up and pay attention!

Charles Van Riper, a well-known speech pathologist and a person who stuttered, also shared some words that shed more light on my fear of stuttering: "The more one stutters, the more he fears certain words and situations. The more he fears the more he stutters. The more he stutters the harder he struggles.

The more he struggles, the more penalties he receives, and the greater becomes his fear."

It was important for me not to read these words from a place of fear, but from a new place of awareness, understanding, and perhaps even acceptance. "Yes, this is how I feel when I stutter." I could never put into words what my fear felt like before, how I really felt when I stuttered.

How does the fear of rejection show up in your life – with certain situations or people, that you view as authority figures? Is there a common thread? Many times, we suppress our feelings of fear because we think if we express who we really are, we won't be accepted or loved. If we suppress our feelings long enough, we get so out of touch with them we don't know they are there or even what they are.

Why do you feel someone knows more about who you are than you do? We've bought into someone else's beliefs. What are some of those beliefs – perfect mother, perfect father, perfect partner, perfect speaker... Just to name a few? What are some of the labels others have put onto you that you have accepted and believed?

So, who is really rejecting you? It's only possible for me to feel rejected when I'm not connected to my wholeness and worth – when I do not realize who I am. I'm the one who is rejecting me! We really don't have any idea what THEY think about us. It's our perception of who we think they think we are (you might want to read that one over a couple of times!)

REALLY IMPORTANT STUFF: What someone thinks about you has nothing to do with who you are, but what *you* think about you does. It has everything to do with who you think you are.

Nothing other people do is because of you. It's because of who they think they are. Even if others insult us, it has nothing to do with us. What they say, what they do and the opinions they give are according to the agreements they've made with themselves. Their point of view comes from who they are, not who you are.

If we react though, then we can probably say "this is about me" – a need to feel safe, to feel accepted and loved. When we don't feel safe in the moment and feel scared, we can ask ourselves

- Do I want to be right?
- Do I want to be in control?

Is it possible that this fear of rejection is arising because of how we are relating to the experience, and not how the experience is relating to us? In that case, it has nothing to do with the other person.

It's important to see the relationship between the thoughts of fear and lack, and how they show up in our lives as experiences, appearing as if someone or something is against us. What is your expectation when you speak; when you go into any situation? Is it fearful? Because our emotions arise from what we make the situation mean.

Here are some ideas to get us beyond the fear of rejection:

- Take one baby step at a time. Know that you do have the courage to step out of your comfort zone.
- Listen to your own feelings of fear, for very often they bring you the answers.
- Be open for the lesson that comes with everything... especially with stuttering.
- Start to take responsibility for how you feel.
- Congratulate yourself! Know that you can love yourself, especially when you stutter.

I was surprised to learn that stuttering could also become my comfort zone. Giving up stuttering can feel like giving up a bad relationship. We know what the relationship is like even if we don't like it, and we stay there because it's what we know. In some ways, it feels safe. The fear of the unknown, what might be expected of us, is greater than the bad relationship or experience we're having.

This might seem strange, but I started to look at what payoffs I might be getting from being a PWS. How many times did I use stuttering as an excuse not to try something new, not to go back to school, not to meet new people? It's important not to look at this this from a place of blame or shame or any of those negative places, but from a place of awareness, and learning, and acceptance.

My greatest fear about stuttering and everything else in my life is that I would not be loved or accepted just as I am. So sometimes I act like who I am not, hoping someone will accept me... I still do that on occasion. I give a small part of me away. For a long time, I didn't realize I was doing this. Because if someone is laughing at me, how can they love me?

The fear was there because I thought who I am isn't good enough, wasn't who somebody else said I should be, or expects me to be. And most important of all who I thought I should be — fluent. Sometimes we spend our whole life not knowing that it is okay to be who we are — kind, compassionate, loveable, and worthy people who stutter. What a difference it makes when we put those positive words and traits in front of the words "people who stutter."

Here is some of the awareness I've gained about fear. Fear is a state of mind. **Fear is a negative thought** that we have about who we are, a situation where our self- esteem is not where it should be.

When I read this definition of fear, suddenly this "thing" that was present every day of my life had a name. It didn't seem so formidable. It didn't seem so hopeless any more.

David Block, a dear friend and member of the CSA, wrote this about the words *Fear is just a negative thought*. "This thing that most of us have that stops us from doing things, this overpowering force that takes control of us, this thing that is so abstract, this thing... now can be something tangible and put into perspective. This thing called 'Fear' is just a negative thought."

Here's a story about facing a fear. It's got nothing to do with stuttering, but one I learned from and applied to stuttering.

I was in Collingwood, Ontario skiing on a hill that I had never skied before. I was standing at the top, looking down at the moguls I would have to go through and around, scared to put my poles in the snow to begin. A friend skied up beside me, and offered this advice to help me traverse this hill and arrive safely at the bottom. He told me to say to myself all the way down the hill, "Moguls are my friends, moguls are my friends."

When I arrived safely at the bottom of the hill, I realized this could also be applied to stuttering, and so my affirmation became "stuttering is my friend." Wow – what a life-changing switch that was! What a difference those words made, and that difference sure didn't happen overnight... another awareness!

There were many new beginnings for me as I was starting to understand what a large part fear was playing in my life. As I began to love and accept myself as a PWS, then my focus on and wish for fluency began to drop away and acceptance of myself as a person who stutters began to take its place. My fear-based thoughts were changing about stuttering and myself!

Here are a few examples of how we can face our fears.

- Take a small risk every day. Make one phone call, and write down what you want to say before you make the call. This is especially helpful when we have a difficult phone call to make.
- Stand beside a stranger at the bus stop, or in a line

anywhere, and just say "Hello" and feel comfortable just saying that. Eventually we can begin "small talk." Feeling emotionally and physically comfortable can come first

- Read *Feel the Fear and Do It Anyway* by Susan Jeffers.

Dr. Carl Scott, a speech pathologist in California, suggests we talk to our fear. He suggests we set our emotions down at a table and get on a first-name basis with them. Ask them why they are in our lives. Ask them what we do to keep them alive. This can be an interesting and informative practice at a support-group meeting.

As a noted speech pathologist, Dr. Joseph Sheehan's main message was "Don't avoid, don't' hide, don't deny your stuttering. The only way you'll ever get over your fear of stuttering and thus become genuinely fluent; is to meet it head-on. Always do the thing you fear, and gradually you will learn not to fear it."

At an NSA conference, I talked with Vivian Sheehan, wife of Dr. Sheehan, who strongly suggested that I practice **voluntary stuttering**. It's about stuttering on purpose, getting stuttering out into the open. When we do this, it takes away the fear and actually gives us the courage to speak again. Instead of focusing on the fear that we're feeling about speaking, we can listen and pay attention to what the other person is saying.

At first, I thought, why would I want to stutter more than I do now? But this practice sure took away a lot of my fear around speaking, particularly to someone on a first-time basis, and is one of the practices I still use today. There's lots of information on the web about this practice.

Dr. Charles Van Riper wrote an article for the NSA newsletter just before he died in 1994. It was his final message, a very powerful one: "Learn to stutter!" It took me a while to accept this one, but I finally felt I might be able to "let it out." I also found out that once I start to face a fear, it starts to disappear, one baby step at a time.

My biggest fear of all was that "they" don't love and appreciate ME... and that still shows up some days. Perhaps there will be some insights and answers in the chapter entitled "Self-Esteem," a very important awareness on our journey to accepting and loving ourselves just the way we are.

CHAPTER 4

____

FEELINGS

My problem was not that I stuttered. It was how I felt about "IT." For many years, I didn't ask myself:

"Are you scared of it? Do you run away from it? Do you feel it is the worst thing that has ever happened to you?" And most important of all, "How do you feel about yourself when you stutter? Is it okay to feel whatever you feel?"

Then I started to understand that I felt embarrassed, angry, worthless at times, and scared most of the time. Fear and anger were two of my worst enemies and because I spent so much time feeling angry and afraid, I wanted and needed to understand these emotions. I hid these feelings away because I didn't know they were there.

As I have learned more about who I am, I'm finding out it's okay to feel the fear that is there because if I don't, it will never go away. PWS have been laughed at, made fun of, and the recipients of stupid jokes and comments. I found it helps me to write about how I feel and what I feel. For me, that is the beginning of being aware.

A book by Leonard Shaw, *Love and Forgiveness*, states there only two emotions — love and fear — and that has always helped me to realize where I am coming from. I invite you to know that it is okay to have these feelings, to acknowledge them, understand where they come from, and then look at some ways to change them, to take charge of them. Only after I started to understand why they are here and from whence they came could I move on from them.

While I was at an NSA conference in San Diego many years ago, I went to a workshop led by Dr. Carl Scott, a speech therapist. He asked us to close our eyes and imagine what fear looked like. I got a picture of a huge dragon-like figure living inside me. Then we were told to ask this picture why it was there. I heard these words loud and clear: "I am here for you to learn from and to grow from." I can still hear them today. In other words, what is here to challenge us is here to grow us emotionally, physically and spiritually. (I'm smiling as I'm writing this and realizing how I still feel this way some days!)

When I was growing up, I can't remember anyone telling me that it was okay to stutter, or if they did, I totally rejected the idea. "It" was never talked about at home and certainly not in school. So I always felt that stuttering was wrong, that I was doing something wrong. I felt I was different, but it wasn't a good different. We can spend our lives thinking about what "they" think about us... and this can apply to so much more than stuttering. I listened to THEM because I thought THEY knew more about who I am than I did. I felt I had to speak better to feel better about whom I am.

Here are some words I wrote many moons ago:

"My feelings are a large part of who I am. To hide my feelings is to hide an important part of who I am. If I run away from my feelings, sooner or later they catch up with me. If I face my feelings and begin to understand them, where they come from, then eventually I will let go of what I want to let go of because I will have no reason to hang on to it any more. I think I'm letting go of my stuttering."

As I'm writing the words "my stuttering," I remember another very important learning experience. I was talking with a coworker at the Conservation Authority where I was working. I spoke about "MY stuttering" and she asked me if I wanted to own it. I think that was the last time I have referred to it as "my" stuttering. Now it's just "stuttering."

I think it's important to have therapy for our emotions as well as stuttering. In a lot of cases, speech therapy looks at the whole person, so therapy for stuttering includes therapy for our feelings. I believe my feelings are a large part of stuttering.

Here's a question I asked myself:

"If I can be fluent when I'm in a room all by myself, why can't I be fluent when I walk out of the room or the door just opens a smidge."

Here's my idea. I can speak fluently in a room all by myself because no one is there to listen to me. I don't have to prove anything to anybody. But when I step out of the room and am speaking to please someone else, once again fearful feelings can take over.

With this awareness in mind, I spent 20 minutes every morning alone in my bedroom reading out loud from Napoleon Hill's book *Think and Grow Rich*. From this experience, I realized there were patterns in my breathing, speech, and sentences that were changing. As a covert stutterer, my sentences were usually very choppy. I would stop in the middle of a sentence; now my sentences were becoming smoother, easier, and I was much more relaxed.

Many moons ago at a conference in New Jersey, I heard these words from Susan Sander, a member of Speak Easy at the time :

"I now know that stuttering has far less to do with speech and so much more to do with fear and courage."

I sat up and paid attention to them. I could relate to these words and was starting to think and understand they were true for me. The acceptance of them and this idea was what was opening up and changing my life in so many ways as a person who stutters. There have been so many people along the way who have shared their insights and truths with me that have changed my life, and for this I am so grateful.

Years ago, I can remember standing in church reading the Bible along with everyone else and noticing that I was not feeling scared and my speech was flowing easily. So I started to imagine that someone else was walking with me, speaking the same words at the same time. And it helped that he was tall, dark, and handsome... (smiling again.)

At a conference in New Jersey, Linda Matthews, a Speech Language Pathologist, said that anxiety is not an emotion we can think our way out of, but an emotion that we have to "DO" our way out of. For example, if we avoid the telephone, we just become more afraid of it. It's so important to congratulate ourselves when we step out and accomplish anything we've been scared to do.

After attending the Bob Proctor seminar in 1989, I went to a seminar by Mark Victor Hansen, a motivational speaker and author. I can still remember watching him move around the stage with such ease. He seemed to be enjoying himself while speaking to so many people. While I was watching him, I got the feeling that I was supposed to be a speaker when I grew up. I turned to my friend Margie and voiced these words:

"Oh My God, I'm supposed to be a speaker when I grow up."

Somehow that made the words real. Two months later, I went to my first Toastmaster meeting and stayed there for five years. They are a wonderful supportive group that changed my life.

Our feelings are a large part of stuttering and who we are. To hide them is to deny an important part of us. I invite you to know that it's okay to feel what you feel. When I run away from my feelings, sooner or later they catch up with me. When I'm aware of them, begin to understand and accept them, then eventually I begin to release them when they no longer serve me. I believe the operative word here is "begin" because for me, this is a lifelong journey of accepting and loving who I am.

I invite you to learn to listen to yourself, to feel the feelings that show up. This can feel scary, and it might help to look for a support group during this time. Here's an idea that our support group did to advertise stuttering and help us move beyond the fearful feelings. Have an "information day" at a local mall. Set up a table and take along information on the NSA, CSA, ISA, etc., as well as your local support group. Stand in front of your table, not behind it, and hand out the information to anyone who is willing to take it. Be aware of the feelings this is bringing up, and congratulate yourself for being with them.

One of the best books I've ever read is *Feel the Fear and Do It Anyway* by Susan Jeffers. This might be a good book to discuss at your support-group meetings.

When someone used to ask me who I was, the first thought that came to my mind was that I stuttered. But now, lots of marvellous things come to mind – I can give them a list – and

somewhere down the line is that I stutter – if it is there at all....
(Once more, I am smiling as I'm writing these words).

One of the most important lessons I've learned is that I am
in charge of how I feel. It is a lesson that still continues. When
I'm angry, it is my own feelings of inadequacy somewhere inside
that make me feel angry. When I feel scared, it is how I feel
about myself inside that makes me feel scared. Nobody makes
me feel anything. I do that all by myself... (darn it!) As our
feelings about who we are get better, when people laugh at us
when we stutter, we can hear that little voice that says "No
matter what you say or do to me, I am still a worthwhile
person." For many years, that was one of my favourite
affirmations. For people to accept us, we first have to accept
ourselves. People feel uncomfortable when we stutter because
we feel uncomfortable. They can read our energy. They can feel
how we feel. I think it's not the other person's responsibility to
make us feel good when we stutter. That is our responsibility.

I also think is it my responsibility to educate my listener
about how I feel when I stutter — sometimes not an easy thing
to do. Have you and I ever thought about how our listener feels
when we are taking two minutes to say something that would
normally take 30 seconds? How do they feel when we block on
a word, sometimes making strange faces and hand gestures?
Have we ever asked them to have patience with us? How do we
expect them to understand when many times we don't
understand?

If we educate the public, maybe someone won't have to go
through what you and I went through; maybe a child in school

will be accepted rather than rejected. Changing is first becoming honest with our feelings. So, I invite you to look at your feelings, begin to understand them and why they are. Talk about feelings at your support group meetings. Most of all, love yourself and have patience with yourself. I believe this will change your whole experience about how you feel about yourself.

CHAPTER 5

SELF-ESTEEM

Stuttering was the beginning of my journey to love and accept myself. It was the reason I began to ask questions about who I thought I was, what stories I was living with and, questioning the feelings I experienced every day of my life. Stuttering can be the start of our journey — because it really is the tip of the iceberg.

I think fluency and accepting ourselves is a holistic happening. It involves our whole being. The first step in the journey and the basis for becoming a whole person is acquiring self esteem . So, what is self-esteem? It's not narcissism that says in essence, "Hey, ain't I enthralling." It isn't bragging: ("look at how great I am.") Self-esteem is the opposite of arrogance: ("I'm better than you are,") and miles apart from self-centeredness: ("the whole world revolves around me.")

Jack Canfield, co-author of the *Chicken Soup for the Soul* series, said, "Self-esteem is made primarily of two things: feeling lovable and feeling capable."

More than anything else, it's being self-forgiving instead of self-condemning and self-respecting instead of self-disgusting.

When you start to love and accept yourself just as you are, you find out what a worthwhile human being you are. You realize that you can have what you need, want or desire (now doesn't that brings up some interesting ideas!).

So, how does a sense of self-esteem help you and me?

1. We realize we are okay just as we are. We don't have to be perfect. Our speech doesn't have to be perfect. Some days, I think I still am a perfectionist because I want everything else in my life to be perfect because my speech wasn't perfect.
2. We'll do things we didn't have the courage to do before, like joining Toastmasters, speaking to people we didn't speak to before, asking for a job we didn't have the courage to ask for before.
3. We won't feel so rotten when we stutter. A little voice inside will say "It's okay" instead of saying, "Screwed up again, didn't you?"
4. Our whole world will change because of how we feel about ourselves. It's like starting all over again. We attract different circumstances into our lives because we *are* different.

We are very special people, usually very intelligent, and certainly very persistent. We have stuttered thousands of times while saying our name, and we still keep on trying. I remember a fellow in our support group who met a young lady in a local bar one night. Instead of telling her his real name, he made one up because he always stuttered on his own name. After going out with her for three months, meeting her family and friends, he had to tell her that his name was not really Ralph after all.

Have you ever used an alias? I know I have. One of mine was Mary Smith...not very creative was it? Let's look at some good that has come into our lives because we stutter. Here are some of my good things:

- Stuttering was the start of loving myself.
- I have met so many incredible brave people.
- I have travelled in Canada, the United States, England, Wales, Germany, Austria, and Belgium to attend and speak at support conferences.
- I have a magnificent obsession. I was so absolutely amazed when I found out there was hope for me as a person who stutters that I want to help people who stutter realize they can accept and love themselves as a person who stutters.
- I have faced my greatest fear, and still do some days, and this has made me realize that I have the courage to face many other fears that might still be lurking.

You might say I could have been someone else or somewhere else if I didn't stutter, but I am very happy where I am and know this is where I am supposed to be. So, as we change our perception, we can change our life. As we start to love and accept ourselves just as we are, this affects many aspects of our lives.

The other chapters in the book are really part of being a whole person, just like self-esteem is, and tie in with this chapter. I have found that they are all a part of who we really are.

CHAPTER 6

SELF-IMAGE

For many moons, I didn't know what self-image meant or how important it is. It's defined in the dictionary as "the idea one has of one's abilities, appearance, and personality." My self-image was of someone who was lacking self-confidence, someone who felt uncomfortable in a group, someone who couldn't ask for what they want in a restaurant. In other words, it was of someone who is not worthy of living a full life, not capable of doing what she wants to do or being who she wants to be.

So to change this, I had to change my self-image so I could have a picture in my mind of what I wanted to be or do.

When I came out of high school, I was hired at The Steel Company of Canada as an experiment because I stuttered. I was glad to get a job, but was very hurt and angry at the same time. Those feelings were there in part because of my self-image. I think I would have taken any job anybody offered me because of who I imagined myself to be. And I worked at Stelco for 30 years — smiling!

A lot of times we scare ourselves rather than motivate ourselves with the pictures in our mind. As an example, let's try a little imagery. Imagine you've been asked to speak at a conference where there are about 500 people. You're standing back-stage, and a man walks out to introduce you. You walk across the stage to the lectern, put your notes down and look out into the audience. They are staring at you, waiting for you to speak. You open your mouth, but you block on the first word. Did you notice something change in your body? What were some of the changes? What did you feel in your body even as you read this?

Now let's look at the same situation from a different perspective.

You've been asked to speak at a conference. There are 500 people in the audience. That's OK because you have been affirming over and over again that to speak to 500 people is no different from speaking to 5 people. In fact, sometimes it's easier because someone in that 500 is going to like you! The same man walks up to the lectern and gives you a wonderful introduction. You walk to the lectern with confidence, look at your audience and see their smiling faces. You begin your presentation saying, "I am so pleased to be here today." How do you feel now? Any different from the first image? You didn't leave your chair, but you imagined two different experiences.

Our body can't tell the difference between a real event and an imagined event. I used to, and still do some days, scare myself by imaging bad pictures about events that haven't even happened. Going to the dentist is one of them! When I imagine bad pictures, I feel the fear as if it is real and then I don't act. It's the response that I imagine that's scaring me, because I feel I can't handle it.

I think this is what happens when PWS are scared to answer the phone – or any situation. We have a picture of the person answering the phone laughing at us or making fun of us that scares us. We're usually thinking about the bad experiences we've had on the phone — not the good ones.

So how about imaging ourselves (having a mental picture of ourselves) of how we want to be? Confident, comfortable in a large group, able to order what we want in a restaurant. I'm thinking of the many meals I've eaten because I ordered what I thought I could say rather than what I really wanted. For years, I drank Molson's beer because I thought it was the only one I could say without stuttering...and I actually grew to like it!

I had, and still have, pictures of who I want to be in my mind. There was a picture of me speaking at a Toastmaster meeting that reinforced doing what I feared the most — speaking in public. So I invite you to see yourself who you really want to be — not who somebody else says you should be or can be. Because the image you have in your mind will affect every part of who you are.

CHAPTER 7

FORGIVENESS: A LIFE JOURNEY

I can't remember the first time I thought about forgiveness or even understood what it was all about, especially how it could be related to my life as a person who stutters. I can't remember anyone in my family, circle of friends, or at work even mentioning the word. But it really came to light for me after reading Gerald Jampolsky's book *Forgiveness: The Greater Healer of All.* This book is responsible for a lot of the thoughts and words that are included in this chapter.

Forgiveness can end the suffering we cause ourselves and others through our judgments — good or bad, right or wrong, should or shouldn't, etc. I invite you to take a look at the many "shoulds" in your life. One of them might be "I should speak fluently, I shouldn't stutter." I'm realizing that we judge others, ourselves, and our experiences just about 99% of the time, and we do this unconsciously. When we make judgments, it's usually a projection of our own guilt and our own judgments of ourselves.

Here was the shocker for me. It really has nothing to do with the other person. "It's the space I'm in – not where they are." It's really how I feel about myself. Usually what I judge someone else for is really what I am judging myself for.

When I don't forgive, this keeps me attached to incidents, people, and experiences that have happened in the past. For example, occasions when people have laughed at us when we stutter. This may have happened many years ago, but we still focus on it, remembering the shame we felt. I still remember a person laughing at me when I was in an elevator in Edmonton at a conference. I can't remember the circumstances or what I said, but I can still hear her laughter when I stuttered. I'm grateful this is an awareness, not something I'm still attached to.

Forgiveness stops our inner battles with ourselves. It allows us to stop recycling anger and blame. Very often, we spend 95% of the day thinking the same things we thought about yesterday. (I can still relate to this.) Forgiveness can change how we see those things, ourselves, and others.

I used to think that if I forgave someone, they had "won." What I was really scared about was that if I forgave them this time, there was a good chance they would hurt me again. Forgiveness is not for the other person — it is for us. It is about us.

"To not forgive is a decision to suffer."

We believe our happiness lies out there, in people, in what is said to us, in experiences that we label as "good." We're looking outside ourselves to find our happiness. We think "this relationship will make me happy, this car will make me happy, this job will make me happy," and perhaps the greatest one of all: "fluency will make me happy." When we search outside ourselves, we can end up feeling frustrated, angry, unhappy, and hopeless.

"Forgiveness is letting go of all hopes for a better past" – one of my favourite quotes in Jampolsky's book.

We will have more peaceful relationships when we stop telling others how to live. I believe this is us wanting to be in control, wanting to be in charge – two experiences that come from a place of fear and for some reason, still show up in my life.

I believe there are only two emotions – love and fear. So that makes it simple for me. I can ask myself: "Am I coming from a place of love, or a place of fear?" Our biggest block to forgiveness is having a belief system that's based on fear, not love. If we can realize this is also true for the other person, this can actually stop us judging them because we know we also go to that place. Forgiveness also means giving up the idea we always have to be right.... This was a big realization for me... and that, my friends, is worth the journey — a journey that still continues for me.

We need to overcome the belief that the past will inevitably repeat itself. How do we do that? By letting go of our guilt and our shame. A big part of forgiveness for me is forgiving myself for all the things I think I should have been; all the things someone else told me I should be and do, accepting their thoughts and ideas for me. (There's that word "should" again!)

It becomes easier to forgive when we choose to no longer believe we are victims. We always have a choice as to what we think, what we say, and how we feel. When we know we have this choice, we can know we are victims no longer. Forgiveness is a continuous process, not something we do just once or twice. It doesn't have to be done in a day, a week, or a year. It is a lifetime journey.

We often hide our anger. That hidden anger becomes what makes it so difficult to forgive. When we start to become aware and acknowledge what we were angry about in the past, we can make the choice to change it.

I can remember taking part in a meditation retreat and hearing the words "sit up straight" and then the words "stay strong" came into my mind. I went into my inner child — Little Mary — who was angry because she felt she had to stay strong when people laughed at her for stuttering. No matter how old we are, there are still experiences to heal from and learn from, if we so desire.

The key term in learning to forgive is "willingness." I am willing to forgive myself and others so I can be happy, healthy, and whole. When you forgive someone, you are not agreeing with or condoning their behavior. It doesn't mean we have to let all people out of jail, we don't have to work for the boss we didn't get along with, or go back to the marriage we left behind.

The forgiveness stage isn't for the other person, it's for you and me. "I forgive you for laughing at me when I stutter." Wow, isn't that a heavy one! But how do you feel when you have forgiven them? It makes us feel good that we've had the guts to say something, first of all. There is a real sense of accomplishment, and our self-esteem goes up a notch. And when our self-esteem starts to improve, we will be able to talk about stuttering.

So something that we thought we were doing for somebody else, we were really doing for ourselves. Knowing this might make it easier to talk to the person about forgiveness. Everyone wants to feel loved and appreciated, and this exercise will help us to feel that way.

Some things we might want to look at: (as I look at the list, I don't think this will be done by lunch time tomorrow... smiling.)

- Forgiving people who have laughed at us.
- Forgiving loved ones who have died.
- Forgiving family members who have not lived up to our expectations — our partners, our mothers, our fathers, our children.
- Forgiving people we work with.
- Forgiving institutions.
- And most of all, forgiving ourselves.

Some stepping stones to forgiveness.

- Be open to the possibility of changing your beliefs about forgiveness.
- Find no value in self-pity — come to know you're not a victim.
- Choose to be happy rather than right — give up control, because you don't have it anyway.
- Look at everyone or everything you meet as your teacher — even stuttering. Some of the people I've forgiven have been my greatest teachers.
- The purpose of forgiveness is not to change the other person, but to change the negative thoughts in our minds, because it's us who suffer.

These words are from Jampolsky on his way to Bosnia in 1998. Words that can apply to each person and every situation:

"It is never too early to forgive.
It is never too late to forgive.
How long does it take to forgive? It depends on
  your belief system.
If you believe it will never happen, it will never
  happen.
If you believe it will take six months, it will take
  six months.
If you believe it will take a second, that's all it
  will take.

*I believe with all my heart that peace will come to
the world when each of us takes the
responsibility of forgiving everyone,
including ourselves, completely."*

This journey is really one baby step at a time. At first, it was easier for me to forgive someone else. No matter how long it takes, it will lead to a journey back home to you. Please know that you are part of a worldwide support group that is here to support you along the way.

CHAPTER 8

AN ATTITUDE OF GRATITUDE

I believe the journey we're on, the life we're living, is about being a whole person and gratitude is an important part to becoming so. There are two parts to this chapter: attitude and gratitude.

First, I looked up "attitude" in the Oxford dictionary and found I could certainly relate to this: "A settled mode of thinking." Attitude is the way I approach things — my point of view. So, then I asked myself: "Do I look at life as an adventure to be enjoyed or as a problem to be solved?" This could certainly relate to stuttering. There are infinite possibilities for living in either adventureland or problemville... and the choice is always ours.

The connection between attitude and altitude is easy to see. If we have a good attitude, our altitude will rise. The reverse is also true. A spiraling attitude goes up or down and can seem to be infinite in either direction. So, how does one get a better attitude? Mine came through reading inspiring books (like those at the end of this book), attending seminars relating to prosperity, gratitude, letting go of fear, spirituality, and just about anything that interested me at the time. I became active in stuttering support organizations – the National Stuttering Association and the Canadian Stuttering Association. These days, there is just about any kind of workshop on line. One I really enjoyed was by Deepak Chopra and Oprah, entitled "Manifesting Grace Through Gratitude" – a 21-day meditation that's free!

Before we move forward, however, it's good to look at some of our roadblocks. One biggie is our attitude toward the past. An important realization is that we can't change the past, but we can change our thoughts about the past. And if we're hanging on to living with how someone has hurt us in the past, let's be aware of this. The chapter on forgiveness gives some insightful information and ways we can begin this journey.

Here's some guidance I received from teachings from Dr. Wayne Dyer.

- I began to look at myself as a recipient rather than a victim. Everything I possess in my life is because of the efforts of others: my computer, my TV, the chair I'm sitting on, the car I'm driving, my apartment, my clothes... and just about everything else. I invite you to look at your own life and make your own list.

Without the efforts of thousands and thousands of people all working in harmony, I would have nothing showing up in my life. Even if we are "self made," we could not have gone past the moment of our independence without the gifts of those very basic items we've used to become selfmade in the first place. I think about the many planes I have flown in to attend conferences and the hotels I have stayed in to attend those conferences; the hundreds of people it takes to get that airplane off the ground, operate the hotel where I stayed, and provide me with meals.

- Practice a silent expression of gratitude when you get up in the morning; when I put my feet on the floor, I say "Good morning, Lord" instead of "Oh, Good Lord, it's morning." Any time you receive a gift — any kind, large or small — when someone calls you, be grateful for every breath you take. These inner reminders to be thankful allow us to be aware of the abundance in our lives, and actually invite more.
- Tell those around you how much you appreciate them. Let your family know how much you love them... smiling when I'm thinking that with my kids, now in their '40s, we still end our conversations with "love you." Say "thank you" to the person who opens the door for you, fills your gas tank, cooks a meal, lets you in line.
- Practice this attitude of gratitude with strangers.

Return a shopping cart to the store rather than leaving it in the parking lot. Pay for the car behind you in the toll booth. I can remember a time when I was on my way to a conference in Buffalo and paid for the car behind me. This still brings a smile and a warm, fuzzy feeling. Send flowers to someone, for no reason. Leave cookies outside someone's door.

- One of the things that changed my life was a gratitude journal. At the end of the day, I listed five things for which I was grateful that day. Even now, I go back and read through individual months or years to help me remember how many times I have been blessed in so many ways.

- Also, be aware of the need to be grateful for the struggles and suffering that are part of life. At times it's easy to be angry at the suffering rather than knowing it is the catalyst for our searching and awakening. Our ability to know the power of love and kindness can grow out of pain and darkness in our past.

So, the big question is, what does/has stuttering taught us? I had never even considered or thought about that question until I attended a conference in Chicago in the late '90s entitled "The Gift of Stuttering." At first, that sure made me sit up and say, "I don't think so." But, as in many times before, my thoughts around this started to change after the conference.

There's a chapter on "The Gift of Stuttering" in this book that is my answer to this question and thoughts around this.

Another step on the gratitude journey is the development of a generous heart; giving of ourselves and all we have manifested without any expectation of anything in return. When we generously share what we receive and move our attention away from what we want, then we receive our greatest gifts.

Generosity teaches us about the inner quality of letting go. Letting go and releasing our attachment is the most freeing thing we can do to liberate ourselves. Needing to hang on to things and money arises out of an inner sense of fear, often feeling incomplete. Practicing generosity aligns us with our sense of completeness and love.

Melody Beattie, author of many books on gratitude, writes, "Gratitude makes sense of our past, brings peace for today, and creates a vision for tomorrow." Wow — that, I believe, is our life journey! I am so grateful for each one of you who has shared your journey with me. There have been many people in many places that I have learned from and laughed with, and for that I will be eternally grateful.

CHAPTER 9

─────────

THE GIFT OF STUTTERING

In the late 1990's, I was asked to speak at a conference in Chicago where the theme was "The Gift of Stuttering." I can remember thinking, *now, what am I going to say about this?* And so I started with the question,

"Is stuttering a gift?"

I realized it had taken a long time — about 60 years — for me to realize it is my gift.

This gift doesn't come wrapped in fancy, shiny paper with a big red bow and lots of sparkles. It comes wrapped in many layers of plain brown wrapping and as we start to peel away the layers — the fear, guilt, anger, and shame — we find that we are the gift, and stuttering is the gift that has opened our eyes to this.

My fear has brought me faith, my anger has brought me patience, my criticism has brought me compassion; not loving me has shown me there is love.

Many years ago, at a conference in Germany, Konrad Schafers said, "Stuttering can be beautiful."

For many years, I rejected this... but that statement stuck with me because it conjures up much hope. I had the nerve to utter these words at a support meeting one night, and from the looks on the group's faces, I knew they thought I had lost it. But at the next meeting, one of our members shared her thoughts about this.

"If, first of all you find out you are beautiful, then you will know that your stuttering is beautiful because it is part of you."

I invite you to consider stuttering as your gift, if you have not already done so, and open the gift to find that you are beautiful...especially when you stutter. As you become aware of who you are, this is what you will share, not only with those who stutter, but with everyone that you meet.

CHAPTER 10

LOVE YOUR BODY & SPIRITUALITY

You might be asking – what is this chapter doing in a book about stuttering? I think it is a part of living a whole and healthy life, of accepting ourselves the way we are. So I invite you to read on....

What is your body for? It's a vehicle for getting the important parts of you around – your heart, your brain, your mind, your feelings, and a lot of very important organs. Don't envy bodies that remind you of a Mercedes Benz – sleek and well put together. I drive a nine-year-old Ford that sure didn't cost what a Mercedes does – but it still gets me where I want to go.

Look for the positive, not the negative. Look for what you have, not what you think you don't have. Concentrate on what works, not on what doesn't. An example of this is the story of Judge Sam Filer of Toronto.

Judge Sam Filer had Lou Gehrig's disease. This terminal neurological illness gradually made the judge a quadriplegic and robbed him of almost all movement. He couldn't walk, talk, or breathe on his own, but he had chosen to live life to the fullest. He went to the court house twice weekly to adjudicate matters in his chambers where the parties didn't have to be present.

He moved in a wheelchair, breathed through a respirator, ate through a feeding tube and tapped Morse code onto an electronic switch that translated the words to a laptop computer with a voice synthesizer. Just image... all that to speak. In an interview, he blinked these words with his eyelids in Morse code, "I am proud to be able to serve my community in my present capacity which in no way impinges on my ability to see, to hear, to think, to read, to reason, and to remember."

Talk about concentrating on what is working for you instead of what is not working! Whenever we get upset because our day isn't going well, let's remember Judge Sam Filer.

When we love and appreciate our body, our body knows it. It will work so much better for us. So, let's take care of it and maintain it. Eat healthy and exercise regularly. (That's what I'm working on these days.) Lead a balanced life – remember to go out to play. We're never too old for recess. Who we are on the inside is much more important than what we are on the outside.

Sometimes we need cookies and milk in the afternoon, and a nap now and then. Ask for a hug if you want one. Author Virginia Satir says that we need four hugs a day for survival, eight hugs a day for maintenance, and twelve hugs a day for growth. Here are six different hugs you can share with your family or your support group....

1. A Frame Hug — You just meet at the shoulders and your butt sticks out a bit.
2. Half-a-Chest Hug — That's self-explanatory.
3. Hip Hug — Your arm usually goes up in the air for this one.
4. Burp-the-Baby Hug — You pat them on the back while you're hugging them. This can mean you're treating them as a child, and stops any emotion. Hmmmmm.
5. Hit-and-Run Hug — Lasts about two seconds because you really don't want to do it.
6. Nurturing Hug — The best kind. You usually ask the other person if it's okay with them.

Loving my body is part of loving myself. You and I are so much more than the outer shell everyone sees. People will start to see some of who we are inside when we know it is there.

HIGHER SELF

There are three levels to a well-balanced life — intellectual, physical, and spiritual. It is important to acknowledge our spirituality, our purpose in life, our higher self. Dr. Wayne Dyer, author of many books, writes, "We are all spiritual beings, having a human experience." However, most of the time, we perceive ourselves the other way around.

As we get in touch with our inner self, our soul, or whatever you call the force that is within each one of us, we will find direction in our lives. What is our purpose in life? What are we here for? As we discover this, we have a focus, a reason for living. It makes decisions about our future a lot easier. It makes life simpler. We will find out we have the ability to be person we choose to be.

CHAPTER 11

———

IT'S NOT REALLY ABOUT STUTTERING

Coming home from an NSA conference in San Diego, I wrote these words:

"This is a journey about finding me. About knowing who I truly am. It's not really about stuttering. The only person who has to love me when I stutter is me."

I knew this was a required journey for me.

One of the major teachings that has helped me is taken from the book, *The Four Agreements* by don Miguel Ruiz. The book is a practical guide to personal freedom, and it asks us to look at the source of our self-limiting beliefs that rob us of joy and create needless suffering. I don't know about you, but I don't want to suffer any more. The second agreement is "**Don't Take Anything Personally**" and I keep going back to this because of the freedom it brings.

If I say I don't like you because your hair is green, you'll probably just laugh. But if I say I don't like you because you're mean and inconsiderate, somewhere inside you might feel this is who you are and react to this. You take it personally because you agree with what's been said. "You should be better, you should look better." And the big one for me was, "You should speak better."

But... Nothing other people do or say is about you or me. It is about who they are and what their beliefs are. Everybody is in a completely different world. Your world isn't the same as mine and mine's not the same as yours, even though we may stutter. Our stories are all different, and our stories change. Very often our "story" is typically one of blame or victimization. It can be some form of "I told you so." This story usually reinforces our sense of identity, who we think we are.

When we take something personally, we assume "they" know who we are and what is in our world. We can feel hurt, offended, rejected, and not loved. We're really setting ourselves up to suffer. We react, many times inside, by defending our beliefs, angry because others haven't accepted us as we are. And the question here is, have *we* accepted ourselves as we are? This is not their responsibility – it is ours. When we no longer have the need to be accepted, whether they laugh with us or at us, we know it has nothing to do with us. It has to do with them and where they are in their journey. Let us recognize and understand this with love in our hearts, without judgment, and without blame.

I can still remember October, 1989, even though it was many years ago. My Dad died, my marriage ended, and my house was sold. Three months later, I went to see my brother in the Florida Keys for some rest, and was reading Louise Hay's book *You Can Heal Your Life* — rather apropos at the time, don't you think!

The third sentence in the first chapter said something like, "I am 100% responsible for who I am, what I am and where I am." I threw the book on the ground because I wanted to blame the breakup on "him," and didn't want to take responsibility for my part or who I was. However, the next morning, I picked the book up and started to reconsider those words, which are still relevant for me today.

Others will always have their own opinions and belief systems about many things — it would be a boring world if they didn't. What they think or believe or feel is not about you and me — it is about who they are and where they are in their journey.

As I look at my own journey many years later, I know — just like stuttering — it's not the actual event that is here for me to learn from. It is the stories I have about it, the feelings I have about it, and the many learnings and blessings that are contained in those stories and feelings.

CHAPTER 12

—————

AND SO MY JOURNEY CONTINUES...

My wish for you is that you wake every morning happy to be alive. May you realize how amazing you are just the way you are.

We are so much more than people who stutter. Expect the best because you are the best, and are worthy of it. We are so persistent. We wake up every day of our lives, with courage to face another day, whether we stutter or not.

For almost 55 years, I spent a lot of evenings sitting on the couch watching TV, scared to join Toastmasters or other groups, because I stuttered. And now I earn my living by speaking.

I invite you to know that you can do whatever you want to do when you take the risks, when you love yourself, when you ask for what you want, and when you know that you are a powerful, loving, human being.

It takes time and energy and perseverance to change our belief systems, and to realize the truth about who we are... and it is worth every single minute. May your life be the amazing life it can be.

Know there are thousands of people who are on the same journey, ready to support you, to reach out to you, and to share this journey with you. You can get in touch with me at dmarywood@yahoo.com. I'd love to hear about your experiences and insights on this journey we share.

Last Request

You most likely picked up this book because of something someone said about it in a "Review" section or word-of-mouth.

If you enjoyed this book or found it helpful, please share your experience with other potential readers.

Help get these life-changing words into more hands.

Please leave an honest review on the platform of your choice (Amazon is one of the most important).

Thank you!

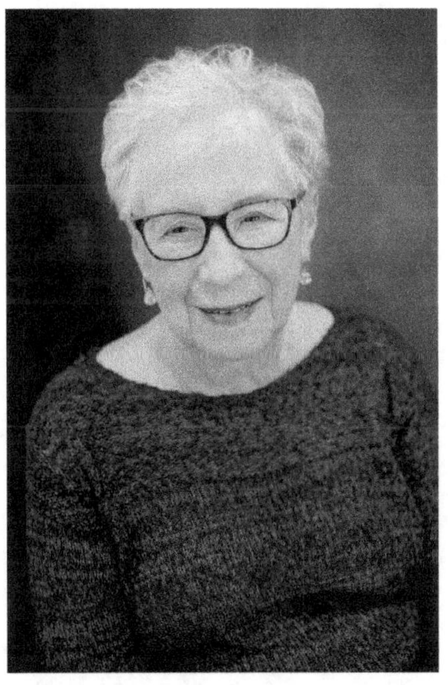

After stuttering for over 50 years, Mary discovered information about the fear of rejection and how it showed up in her life as a person who stutters. She knew this was an important part of her journey that would bring change. As her journey continued, Mary began focusing on accepting herself as a person who stutters—still her focus today—rather than fluency which had always been her goal. Mary first attended a conference for people who stutter in Ottawa in 1993 where she presented a workshop on self-esteem. Since then, Mary has inspired people at conferences in Canada, the United States, parts of Europe, and Great Britain. In 2005, she was ordained as a Unity minister, a lesson that taught her you never know what's around the next corner. After serving at churches in Fort Wayne, Indiana and Mississauga, Ontario, Mary is now looking forward to retirement—whatever that means—and what surprises it will bring.

Feel free to reach out to Mary at dmarywood@yahoo.com.

RESOURCES

- *You Can Heal Your Life:* Louise Hay
- *As a Man Thinketh:* James Allen
- *The Power of Positive Thinking:* Norman Vincent Peale, 1952-90, Ballantine Books
- *Love & Forgiveness:* Leonard Shaw, 2989, Self-published
- *Feel the Fear and Do It Anyway:* Susan Jeffers, 1987, Ballantine Books
- *The Magic of Believing:* Claude Brtistol
- *What to Say When You Talk to Yourself:* Shad Helmstetter, 1982, Grindle Press

- *Change Your Mind, Change Your Life:* Jampolsky & Cirincione, 1994, Bantam
- *Man's Search for Meaning:* Victor E. Frankl, 1984, Beacon Press
- *Psycho-Cybernetics:* Maxwell Maltz, 1960, Prentice-Hall
- *Manifest Your Destiny:* Wayne Dyer, 1997, Harper & Collins

*affiliate links through Amazon Associates go towards the book production and marketing